PRESCRIPTION COMEDY

AN UNLIKELY ANTIDOTE TO PHYSICIAN BURNOUT

PRANATHI KONDAPANENI, MD, MPH.

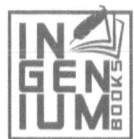

CONTENTS

Introduction   1

THE WHITE COAT'S FAILURE

1. Dent in My Armor   7
2. Anatomy of Disillusion   13
3. Anatomy of Physician Burnout   19
4. Female Physician Burnout   25
5. Why Physicians Burn Out   27
6. The Burnout Cure   33

MY COMEDIC ADVENTURES

7. The Flame Challenge   39
8. Zip Zap Zop   45
9. The Connection Conundrum   51
10. Foreign Accents   57
11. Educate, Entertain, Inspire   65

THE COMEDIC CURE

12. The Good of a Simple Smile   73
13. Jump. Dance. Treasure.   79
14. A Beautiful Goodbye   83

APPENDIX   87
Acknowledgments   89
About the Author   91
Other books by Pranathi: 93
Notes   95

Copyright @2021 Pranathi Kondapaneni

All rights reserved in all countries and territories.

Published by Ingenium Books Publishing Inc.

Toronto, Ontario, Canada M6P 1Z2

https://ingeniumbooks.com

Ingenium Books supports copyright. Copyright fuels innovation and creativity, encourages diverse voices, promotes free speech, and helps create vibrant culture. Thank you for purchasing an authorized edition of this book and for complying with copyright laws by not reproducing, scanning, or distributing this book or any part of it without permission. You are supporting writers and helping ensure Ingenium Books can continue to publish nonfiction books for readers like you. You are permitted to excerpt brief quotations in a review. For all other permission requests, please contact the author in writing via the contact form at www.thephysicianphoenix.com.

ISBNs:
978-1-989059-17-3 (paperback/softcover)
978-1-989059-18-0 (electronic)
978-1-989059-19-7 (hardcover/hardback)
978-1-989059-21-0 (audiobook)
978-1-989059-20-3 (large print)

This publication was written by a physician. Material in this book is for education and entertainment purposes only and is not to be misconstrued as medical advice. The reader has no therapeutic relationship with the physician author. While the publisher and author have made every attempt to verify that the information provided in this book is correct and up to date, the publisher and author assume no responsibility for an error, inaccuracy, or omission.

"The human race has one really effective weapon, and that is laughter."

MARK TWAIN

*To my **parents**, for giving me wings.*
*To my **teachers**, for gifting me comedy.*
*To **Thanhvan**, for granting me courage.*

INTRODUCTION

WHITE AS A CLOUD on a full sunny day.

Crisp as a freshly-laundered sheet.

Pure as the touch of a newborn.

These were the sensations that washed over me as I felt the edges of my new white coat, which had just been given to me in the White Coat Ceremony. It was the autumn of 1997. It was just a short white coat because I was still a medical student. Still, it was exhilarating to feel the material, smell the freshness, and see my name in cursive blue above the right breast pocket. This was my first step on the path toward mending, healing, and curing. Or so I thought.

During the ceremony, the first-year medical students were inducted into the world of medicine by reciting the Hippocratic oath. The line that resonated with me the most was the following: "I will remember that there is art to medicine as well as science, and that warmth, sympathy, and understanding may outweigh the surgeon's knife or the chemist's drug."[1]

When I look back on that day, I remember feeling a sense of innocent, optimistic empowerment. Over the years, this sense of empowerment would be replaced by realistic, pessimistic downtrodden-ness. Before medical school, I had envisioned a Norman Rockwell–painting utopia in which doctors spent time connecting with patients. Instead, the reality was a George Orwell–flavored dystopia in which doctors were cogs in a machine with no decent time for connecting with patients.

As the weight of a medical system that didn't value connection grew, my burnout festered like an open sore. The pus of feeling like a glorified bookkeeper in a system of endless paperwork and non-patient-related tasks oozed out of me slowly, day by day. What could I do about the situation? I couldn't change a healthcare system that valued perverse economic health incentives over patient care. Yet, I could improve the communication inside my own clinical office. Thus began my quest to improve the physician-patient bond through improved communication. Little did I know that my answer would be found in the world of comedy.

So, did I become a professional comedian? Nope. And that's ok. Because that was never my goal. Frankly, I'm pretty hooked. What I garnered from my comedic education was more than I could have expected. At its heart, the true beauty of comedy isn't in making people laugh but in connecting with an audience.

Comedy proved to be not just a communication exercise but a healing one. What started out as a journey to improve communication within an office setting became a much deeper journey toward healing a burned-out shell of a physician. While I may not be a professional comedian or a renowned physician coach, I sincerely believe that in sharing my journey, I can help my fellow physicians who feel downtrodden, disenfranchised, and disenchanted by the weight of this medical system. Unless one has walked in the shoes of a shattered physician, it's hard to understand the swamp which can swallow a physician whole.

Physicians are a particular breed. Many people see us as lucky because our job provides a stable, decent income. But we ultimately carry the burden of treating a human being's most precious resource: health. Couple this responsibility with a broken healthcare system—physicians face a hefty load indeed.

In the first section of this book, we'll delve into physician burnout. First, I'll relate my personal loss of faith in medicine. Then, we'll look at the greater burden of burnout within the overall community of physicians. I used to think I was singular in my affliction. However, I later learned that physician burnout is rampant.

In the second section of the book, I'll share my comedy journey, as I wandered from a simple writing competition into improvisation, stand-up comedy, and comedic writing. Given that I'm a reserved introvert, my travels through comedy stretched me further than I could have imagined.

In the final section of the book, we'll look at the everlasting imprints my comedic travels left on me. I want to impart to my fellow healthcare providers the lessons that helped me defeat burnout.

Overall, in this book I've concentrated on the overarching experiences and education I gathered during my comedic journey. There were also many practical lessons learned.

So, let's begin down the path on which comedy and medicine intertwine to heal the healer.

THE WHITE COAT'S FAILURE

SECTION ONE

1. DENT IN MY ARMOR

Our life is made by the death of others.

LEONARDO DA VINCI

PITTER. Patter. Splat.
Pitter. Patter. Splat.
Pitter. Patter. Splat.

Pitter went the raindrops against the window ledge. Patter went the hospital bed's wheels. Splat went the blood onto the floor of the intensive care unit (ICU). Twenty-four years old and recently graduated from medical school, these were the sounds that greeted me daily during my intern year. My short white student coat had been replaced with a *proper* long white coat. I wore it with pride.

After a busy evening in the emergency room, like a sheriff making rounds in a prison, I made early morning rounds through my patient charts. At the nurse's station, I munched on popcorn and flipped through my to-do list. So long as the charts were covered, the nurses' questions were answered, and the labs all checked out, I could rendezvous with the vending machine for my late-night sustenance. Then I could go to sleep. After all, it wasn't as though the ICU patients would bug me—most were in a coma, or at least heavily sedated.

Everything seemed to be in order, so I decided to get my dinner. I had long ago missed the chance to consume the cafeteria's particle board. It wasn't a great culinary loss. After all, the hospital cafeteria's job was to keep the hospital in business by serving coronary-plugging delicacies such as fried-cheese sandwiches. Alas, an admission to the ICU sent my much-anticipated vending-machine-dinner plans awry.

The hospital admission had started routinely enough.

Order the lab work.

Order the medications.

Order the hairbrush . . . ?

The patient was a silver-haired, green-eyed granny, and she was sitting upright in the bed in her room. Next to her sat a raspy-voiced, mischievous-eyed granddaddy. In the middle of a giggle fest, Granny and Granddaddy looked up and smiled at me as I entered. It was unusual to see the living in the land of the ICU. This contrast was made even more stark by the couple's infectious laughter lighting up the room.

Granny was well within the land of the living but had been admitted to the ICU for close cardiac observation. The regular intermediate cardiac care unit was full. Therefore, this ICU bed was being used as an overflow bed. Granny was to stay overnight for monitoring until a cardiac patient was discharged the next day.

She'd been suffering from heart palpitations. Over the last two days, her heartbeat had fluttered back and forth between fast and slow. I asked her, "Why didn't you get help two days ago?" "How could I tell, dear?" she replied with a wicked grin. "Around my husband, my heart is always aflutter with butterflies." As these lovebirds teased and smiled at each other, I couldn't help but be amazed by the beauty of their obvious love within the ICU's gray harshness. I documented the time of the interview: 2:36 a.m.

An hour later, her heart would be aflutter no more.

ABOUT A QUARTER of an hour after I concluded the patient's history and physical interview, the monitoring alarms went off like fire engine sirens throughout the whole ICU. Medical staff rushed into Granny's room to find she had pulled her monitoring leads off. She apologized for causing such a fuss. She'd pulled off all the leads to go to the bathroom, coif her hair, and apply her makeup. The hospital gown was hideous enough, she said—she wasn't going to spend the rest of the night without a little lip gloss and neatly parted hair.

A patient setting off the screaming ICU alarms is quite a bit more effective than caffeine for waking up sleepy hospital staff. After entering the room and learning the reason for the disturbance, I was a bit peeved at first. But as Granny pleaded her case, I relented. Her grooming before saying good night to her husband had been a nightly ritual for over forty years of marriage. She pleaded for ten to fifteen more minutes of grooming time before getting hooked up to all the monitors again. This spry granny already looked sophisticated enough to grace the cover of a silver-fox fashion magazine—especially compared to my current Bride-of-Frankenstein appearance, due to the busy on-call day. I gave in. What was the harm in ten to fifteen more minutes of primping? She agreed to get back into bed and not remove the monitoring leads again afterward. My stomach was growling and my calves were aching. Who was I to get in the way?

After I completed all the paperwork, I was finally ready to head down to my vending-machine-dinner rendezvous. But the fire-station alarms blasted off again. I groaned. What was it this time? Mascara?

But it wasn't an issue of makeup. It was a deadly heart arrhythmia. As soon as Granny's monitoring leads had been reapplied, the alarm bells had begun screaming incessantly. Granny was sitting up and watching the commotion with a smile of inquiring amusement. Her husband was quickly ushered out of the room.

Within one minute, the cardiac code protocol flew into action.

Within two minutes, Granny slipped into a coma.

Within three minutes, Granny's heart stopped.

For over thirty minutes we worked to bring light back into those olive eyes. Chest compression after chest compression. I couldn't let her go like this. I wouldn't let her go like this. Chest compression after chest compression. I kept trying to pump warmth back into her pale skin. Chest compression after chest compression. Finally, my senior resident grabbed my hands and said, "Enough. Time to call it."

The time of a heart no longer aflutter: 3:48 a.m.

As the cardiac monitors were turned off, I stood there for what felt like an eternity looking at the clock. My resident's beeper awoke me out of my trance. He had to rush down to the emergency room to take care of another urgent patient. So, I was left to deal with the death note. I wrote it mechanically, in the corner of the room, while nurses cleaned up the mess. After Granny looked presentable, I went out to talk to Granddaddy. As he listened, the flames in his eyes turned to embers, then flickers, and finally ashes.

Granddaddy reentered the room at 4:19 a.m. His incredulous gaze pierced my core. Slowly, he touched her hands. Slowly, he stroked her forehead. Slowly, he pulled down her eyelashes. Slowly, guilt seeped through my skin. Slowly, my heart sank. Slowly, a chill settled into my bones.

Intellectually, I knew there was nothing more we could have done. We had responded within minutes. Yet, our best efforts had failed us miserably. In that moment, as I absorbed this man's tears, intellectuality couldn't penetrate my heart.

As I watched Granddaddy say goodbye to his beloved, I kept

going over the night's events again and again in my mind. All I could feel was guilt. Guilt for letting Granny do her makeup for ten to fifteen minutes. Guilt for getting irritated the second time the fire-station alarms screamed. Guilt that her heart would never be aflutter with butterflies around her husband anymore.

In the preceding years, I had witnessed death on numerous occasions. However, this was the first time a patient had unexpectedly died under my direct watch. She'd been so alive. She'd come in for a routine overnight admission. She wasn't supposed to die.

Just as the warmth of a lover's first surprise kiss always resides within one's heart, the chill of a doctor's first surprise death always resides within one's bones.

A few minutes later, my pager went off. It was the emergency room. Another admission. I looked up at the clock. It was 5:16 a.m. My vending-machine-dinner rendezvous would have to wait. It was time to get back into doctor-machine mode and help the next patient.

Before this mode took over completely, I looked down at my crumpled-up white coat. Granddaddy had just lost the love of his life. Nurses and physicians were whizzing around him attending to other patients. ICU alarm bells were screeching like fingernails on a chalkboard. In the midst of this cacophony, this poor man was trying to hold back tears. Instead of giving him the time he deserved to ask questions, I had to give him curt answers and rush off to the next admission.

The first dent in my white coat of armor was already beginning to show.

2. ANATOMY OF DISILLUSION

GRANNY'S DEATH had penetrated my white coat of armor. But in that moment, I wasn't aware of the consequences. I was too busy being the doctor. It wasn't until I knitted the pieces of my disillusionment together over a decade later that I realized that night had been the turning point.

At every stage of my medical training (medical school, internship, residency, fellowship, etc.), I convinced myself things would get better as time went on. But instead of being filled with mending, healing, and curing, my days were filled with paperwork, scut work, and stupid work. Once I reached attendinghood, which is full-on medical practice after all medical training has been completed, there were no further training ladders to climb. There were no further arguments I could make that life as a physician would get better. There were no further disillusionment charms to cast. The hope illuminated by the white coat had been false.

To be fair to the white coat, I'd entered medical school without doing my research. I was accepted to medical school at sixteen years of age. At seventeen, I entered a seven-year combined program. In seven years, I obtained two undergraduate degrees in economics and biology, a medical degree, and a master's degree in public health. On stage during my medical-school graduation, at the age of twenty-four, instead of feeling elated, I felt nauseous. The path didn't feel right. But I ignored my inner voice.

At twenty-eight, I finished a neurology residency and decided to take a year off to travel. I'd already been accepted into a fellowship, which would start after my year off. I'd specifically chosen this fellowship because it was run by a well-known neurologist who did research on pregnant women and epilepsy. I knew that doing a research project in an area of my academic interest would help me secure an academic job focused on treating women with epilepsy. The path ahead of me was perfectly linear. And had I not taken that year off, I would have gone down this perfectly laid-out route.

During my travel year, I got thrown off a train while searching for the Pilsner factory in the Czech Republic, witnessed the screaming of a child in the midst of a seizure due to a hot-water trigger (hot-water epilepsy), and caressed the face of a tearful acid-burn victim. A flame had been sparked. The constraints of the perfectly crisp white coat began to fritter. Yet, it would be many more years before the white coat's disillusionment charms would finally be broken for good.

I continued to travel one or two times a year, either around the United States or abroad. What I loved the most about travel was hearing, feeling, and seeing the stories of regular people in their natural habitats. This love of story was also what sustained me in medicine. The stories of my patients, their trials and tribulations, the beauty of the human experience kept my flame slightly a-flicker.

Trapped by a good life, I continued in clinical medicine for more than a decade. I started my first attending job in December 2008. A stable paycheck allowed me to buy an apartment, travel abroad, and save for the future. Inside, however, I was dying a slow death. The only drops of water in the barren desert were my patients' stories. But as the onerous medical system allowed less and less connection over the years, these drops of water slowly dried up.

In the summer of 2012, my disenchantment with medicine worsened. My workplace experience was going downhill due to a chief operating officer who had little organizational skills and employees who were suffering the result of her incredible incompetence. Two of my favorite staff members left within a few months of each other. Then, a third office-staff member was fired for speaking up regarding patient complaints. At this point, I handed in my three months' notice.

After I handed in my resignation, the administration became belligerent and began withholding salary. I held on for as long as I could. A month and a half later, on the advice of my lawyer, I left the toxic situation. Before leaving, I explained in detail the major patient issues to the remaining physician in order to facilitate transfer of care. My patients had always been my top priority, despite the administration antics. I just wanted to move forward and put the whole matter behind me.

I then took on a self-employed position in which I contracted with a sleep laboratory—I paid rent to the facility, where I saw patients and read studies. I billed for my own consultations and sleep -study interpretations. In my first job, my appointment slots were thirty minutes for new patients and fifteen minutes for return patients, as mandated by the CEO (to create more revenue). At the sleep laboratory, I extended the slots: thirty minutes for return patients and forty-five minutes for new patients. Eventually, I had to cut down the new-patient appointments to thirty minutes as well, at the request of the administrator. But at least the return-patient visits were twice as long as they were in my previous position, and I wasn't dependent on someone else for my paycheck.

Eventually, market forces started to put pressure on the sleep laboratory, as they had been doing in the medical field in general. Due to decreasing compensation for and increasing barriers to testing—a result of prior authorizations of sleep studies coupled with the rise of cheaper home-sleep-study testing—this sleep laboratory began to suffer in earnest in late 2015. Administrators tried to compensate for the loss of revenue by increasing the volume of sleep studies, but this was a losing game. Patient care and communication deteriorated, and the staff grew weary. I left this position in the spring of 2018.

Since 2014, patient out-of-pocket costs have been increasing. These costs include co-pays, deductibles, co-insurance, and premiums. Even though I'm a physician, it was hard for me to make heads or tails of the insurance statements my patients showed me. When a patient complained to me of hardship, I tried my best to give them a break. If they asked for a cheaper alternative or wanted to spread out appointments, I tried my best to help them out. Yet no matter how often I told patients I had no control over their deductibles, premiums, or other insurance matters, I was the one to blame. And if the sleep laboratory staff didn't get proper prior authorizations for procedures, the patients would get angry with me. In addition, when front office staff told the patients that this sleep facility or the sleep physician was in their health insurance network (when in fact the facility or physician were out of the patient's health insurance network), the patients would get mad at me over the extra cost of an out-of-network visit. No matter who was to blame or what went wrong, I would get yelled at—because the physician is the face of all that's wrong in medicine.

Many patients think physicians have more knowledge about or power over insurance than we actually do. We don't know what drugs are cheaper under your specific insurance plan unless you tell us. We don't know if your deductible is met. We don't know if you're in or out of network.

While I empathized with and tried to help most patients, if they were at least civil with me and took the time to explain their situation, I had no sympathy for patients who were outright disrespectful. While most patients are good people, there are always a few who just aren't decent. Physicians who abuse their power and mistreat patients should certainly be held accountable, but what about patients who mistreat physicians? On numerous occasions I've been called a fucking dip-shit or a bitch when disagreeing with patients or confronting them on issues such as questionable medication usage.

Administrators would push back when I asked patients behaving in sexually inappropriate ways to be removed from my clinic and transferred to another physician. While the administration was sympathetic to my cause, no one wanted to anger the patient—because the patient was the customer. I will put up with a lot, but I have my limits, and eventually I pushed back. Over the course of five years, I asked for three patients to be removed: one who tried to grab my behind, one who kept asking me out on dates, and one who tried to record a video of my breasts with his cell phone.

In early 2015, in a bid to improve my work situation, I ventured out to learn about communication. While I couldn't make things better with every patient, I could at least try to help the patients who were decent to me. During patient visits, I was spending more time on insurance questions and less time on medical issues. Therefore, it was even more crucial for me to communicate with the patient in an efficient manner.

These were the steps that led me to explore standup comedy.

But first, I had to learn about physician burnout.

3. ANATOMY OF PHYSICIAN BURNOUT

PHYSICIAN BURNOUT IS A HIDDEN EPIDEMIC. In his 2013 TEDMED talk, Dr. Zubin Damania said, "When I looked in the mirror, all I saw was a burned-out, disconnected zombie with a stethoscope covered in bacteria."[1] Dr. Damania, who practiced medicine in California, went on to describe what used to be his typical day: tackling mounds of paperwork, taking endless calls from administrators, dealing with colleagues asking him to do more with less, responding to constant messages, taking care of sick patients, and dealing with an infuriating electronic medical system. Sound familiar? It does to me.

Dr. Damania also discussed the issue of not being present for his family after his workday. During my attendinghood years, I felt so drained by patients, office staff, and administration that the idea of trying to be present for friends and family was somewhat of a joke. Often, after a workday, all I wanted was to retreat to a place of peace and quiet. Dr. Damania noted that he'd become a zombie with a stethoscope. I, a neurologist by training, had become a zombie with a reflex hammer.

Though Damania's talk was given in 2013, its relevance has unfortunately only grown. In the United States in particular, the worsening healthcare system has created a new crop of burned out physicians who go through their jobs in a mechanical fashion. Given skyrocketing healthcare costs and decreasing revenue, physicians in the United States are being asked to do more and more with less and less.

According to Medscape's *National Physician Burnout and Depression Report 2018*, forty-two percent of physicians reported burnout. The highest rate of burnout was for physicians forty-five to fifty-four years of age. The largest contributors to burnout were bureaucratic tasks (fifty-six percent) and lack of respect from patients (sixteen percent).[2] Forty-eight percent of females and thirty-eight percent of males reported burnout.

What is Burnout?

Throughout my medical career I've talked with many colleagues about burnout, and in physician circles, how it manifests is well-known: extreme exhaustion, compassion fatigue, and efficacy concerns.

Extreme exhaustion: This includes physical and emotional exhaustion. The physician simply cannot take on another task or make another decision. They may feel as if they're dragging themselves through concrete and just want this heavy weight to lift.

Compassion fatigue: Rarely does a physician go into medicine without an underlying compassion for patients. However, when a physician is burned out, they no longer have the emotional capacity to be present for patients or loved ones.

Efficacy concerns: Being a physician is a very hard job that requires constant vigilance. And this job is made even harder when the physician is unsure of their purpose. Is it to help patients or fill out insurance forms? Is it to help patients or answer the administrator's questions? Is it to help patients or catch up on billing paperwork? If and when a physician loses faith in the guiding light—helping the patient—then the very purpose of their job can be called into question: What am I doing here? Do I really make a difference? Do I really help people?

Christina Maslach, in her book *The Truth About Burnout*, described burnout as an erosion of the soul caused by a deterioration of one's values, dignity, spirit, and will.[3]

Burnout and Patient Communication

Physicians are often trying to get a lot of information across in a timely and concise manner. That's why we have standardized methods of communication—the SOAP note, for example. The first part of the note describes a patient's subjective complaint. The next part of the note describes objective things such as vital signs, physical exam findings, and laboratory tests. The next part outlines the medical assessment of the patient based on the subjective and objective findings. Finally, the note details a plan with steps to be taken. These notes are often filled with jargon and abbreviations.

If you phone a consultant to ask for an opinion on a patient, you need to convey complex material quickly and succinctly using a recognized format of communication. This allows the consultant to ask the right questions and form a reasonable opinion. This medical-staff-to-medical-staff communication serves a specific purpose and is meant to be technical, not conversational. But what happens when this boring, jargon-filled, technical language overflows into conversations with patients?

The Car Mechanic and the Physician

I have no expertise in car maintenance. Nor do I have any interest in learning about it. When I take my car in for an oil change, the technician often rattles on about the different types of oil, what needs to be changed, maintenance recommendations, etcetera. Normally, I simply ask them to do what they did last time, and my cars tend to last for many years. Truth be told, I don't understand much of what they say. Thankfully, whenever I've had an issue with a vehicle, someone was able to translate car speak for me. But if I feel this unsure about basic car maintenance due to a lack of understanding of *car speak*, how must *doctor speak* make a vulnerable patient feel?

I believe most physicians do care and try their best to translate *doctor speak* for the patient. But with the current rate of burnout in the physician community, it's easy for physicians to slip into doctor speak. If a physician is experiencing burnout, they may not have the energy, emotional reserves, or confidence to avoid *doctor speak*. As a result, the patient may not understand their medical condition fully and may also feel that the physician isn't relatable. This can lead to poorer health outcomes and decreased patient satisfaction, which in turn can put more pressure on the physician to perform. Hence, the burnout worsens and a vicious cycle ensues.

When Burnout Becomes More Than Just Burnout

It's often difficult to know when burnout isn't just burnout but something more serious, such as depression. According to the Medscape report, fifteen percent of physicians stated they had depression.[4]

Physicians tend to take on too much and put the needs of others ahead of their own. They don't like to admit weakness. I often wonder if the rate of depression is actually higher than what's stated, and if, in some cases, it's more severe than the physician lets on.

There are physicians who move on from depression to suicide. The morbid joke within the medical community is that *every year, a graduating class gets to go on to graduate forever.* In other words, the number of physicians who commit suicide each year is around the same as the number of students in an average graduating medical-school class.

Dr. Pamela Wible is a primary care physician who in 2015 gave a TEDMED talk about physician suicide. Having collected hundreds of suicide letters from physicians, she discussed the reasons why physicians kill themselves. These reasons include untreated depression, soul-crushing medical training, bullying, sleep deprivation, PTSD due to medical school, improper medical licensing board rules, lack of privacy regarding medical data, painful schedules, assembly-line jobs, and an inability to feel human due to the sheer stress of medicine. Dr. Wible noted that each year, one million patients lose their doctors to suicide.[5]

I still remember the first day of medical school. We were such a bright and cheerful bunch. So idealistic. It's tragic that people who go into a profession to help others often end up hurting themselves.

4. FEMALE PHYSICIAN BURNOUT

IT DIDN'T SURPRISE me to learn that women physicians have a higher burnout rate than their male counterparts. And women tend to manifest burnout differently than men. One study shows that female physicians are more likely to express all three symptoms, whereas men are more likely to display extreme exhaustion and compassion fatigue and less likely to have efficacy concerns.[1]

There are deeply rooted reasons at play within our society as to why burnout affects women more than men. Women tend to be treated differently by subordinate staff. Time and time again, I've witnessed how staff react when given a task by a female physician and when given the same task by a male physician. A male doctor who asks why a task hasn't been done is seen as vigilant. The female doctor in the same scenario is bossy.

And the subordinates often treat the female physicians differently. Some of my male subordinates have directly resisted my authority—they've tried not to call me "doctor," they've tried flirting with me to get out of responsibility for a mistake, they've called me inappropriate names, and they've blatantly not performed tasks. The male subordinate's psyche seems focused on power. Overall, male subordinates seem more comfortable with the power hierarchy than female subordinates, but they don't necessarily accept the female physician's place within that hierarchy.

Women, on the other hand, tend to prefer an equal playing field. Therefore, female subordinates often want to pull their female superiors down to their level. Sometimes the behavior is blatant (not performing a task, for example). But often it's more indirect. One female staff member wondered why I wouldn't accept the advances of a patient who was asking me out ("at least you could get a date," she said), and another overreacted when I asked her why a chart wasn't in my box while a patient was waiting (according to her, I had a "tone").

Over the years, I've learned not to take these slights personally. They say more about the offender's issues than my own. Instead, I choose to keep my distance from these sorts of people and to keep my work life strictly about work. There's enough negativity in life without this kind of drama.

The behaviors of administrators also play a part in female physician burnout. For example, a colleague of mine once came into the middle of the technician room and drew a picture of buttocks on the whiteboard. He announced that if a patient was an asshole, he'd draw this picture in their chart. The staff laughed at this. I thought it was highly inappropriate. And if I'd done the same thing, I believe I would have gotten a severe rebuke.

One of my patients told me he always saw female physicians whenever possible. I asked him why, and he replied, "Because women always want to mother and please people, so they'll take care of me better."

While society is changing, there are still very different expectations of women. Many of the MomMD blogs discuss the burden that women place on themselves to be the perfect caretakers and to please others.[2] When this need to be a people-pleasing, perfect caretaker is paired with the stress of medicine, the result is a hefty burden.

5. WHY PHYSICIANS BURN OUT

THERE ARE several contributing factors that lead to physician burnout, including culture, conditioning, and environment. Let's start with the conditioning we receive in medical school.

Medical Training Mentalities

Physicians in the United States must endure a minimum of seven years of training to become attendings (four years of medical school and three years of residency). When physicians are inducted into medical school with the white coat, we enter a world in which we're taught that we're different. We're taught that we have special powers—we can perform complex medical duties on a few hours of sleep, for example.

After all, we physicians are different. We physicians are special. We physicians have a white coat of armor.

Medical school and residency foster an unhealthy culture. For example, the attending physician will often quiz medical students and residents using the Socratic method until they can no longer answer any questions. This normally doesn't make the medical professional feel smart, only stupid. As well, senior residents tend to give lower-level residents unwanted tasks. Lower-level residents then pass these tasks down to medical students when they can. The lower-level resident or medical student does what's asked because one should never show any sign of weakness. Medical training involves a fair amount of bullying and hazing, and these behaviors often go unquestioned.

It takes a particular type of person to get through medical school and medical residency: a hardworking, vigilant, independent thinker who can deal with the high risks that come with taking care of a patient's health. However, this work-environment mindset can also set the physician up to become a workaholic, perfectionistic loner over the long term.

The Post-Training Environment

Sometimes the job environment itself can be the trigger. Maybe the clinic is poorly run, your boss doesn't know what they're doing, the hospital politics are childish, your colleagues are petty, you don't get paid properly, the call schedule is too strenuous—the list goes on and on.

Often, administrators make changes without the input of the physician. In early 2009, the administrator decided that my office should be rearranged, and my desk and chair were repositioned. The only little problem was that afterward, I couldn't physically get around the desk to sit in my chair. No one noticed this until I got to the clinic. It took an hour to sort things out, and the first patient was kept waiting for forty-five minutes.

Since I started as an attending over a decade ago, physicians have seen only more administrative paperwork and insurance-related phone calls. It seems as though we're now documenting things to meet regulation requirements or for billing purposes instead of for the purpose of transferring medical knowledge to help the patient. For example, how many physicians really think the review-of-systems questionnaire—a specific set of medical questions physicians are taught to ask under certain conditions—is relevant? Yes, it's important to know how to ask the review-of-systems questions when needed. But the reality is that the documentation of the review of systems mainly exists as a requirement for regulation/billing purposes.

Systems that were designed to help physicians are often detrimental to them. Electronic medical records are a good example. Given my poor handwriting, I'm all for typed-up medical records, and in the past, physicians could dictate these records to a human transcriptionist. But today, in order to save costs, physicians are forced to dictate their notes into a computer directly or type them up themselves. Given that they have a limited amount of time, most of their attention is focused on the medicine instead of catching typos in a note—understandably so.

The computer acts as a barrier between the patient and the physician, preventing communication. And don't get me started on the clicks. I've never understood why it takes so many clicks in an electronic medical record to do something as simple as order a referral. More clicks equals less time with the patient and more frustration for the physician.

I have hope that the issues with electronic medical records will change in the near future as a result of technology. Imagine a day where physicians don't have to type up notes because a voice-activated electronic medical system automatically does it for them. This would be a good thing, as long as the administration designs the system with physician input.

Lack of Self-Care

"The patient always comes first" is a mantra in medical school. If I got a penny every time I heard this throughout medical school, residency, and fellowship, I would easily be a millionaire! Now, before anyone gets up in arms, I'm not saying that the patient isn't important. I'm saying that the patient shouldn't become so important that the physician's well-being suffers.

Whenever you board an airplane, you're reminded that in the event of an emergency, you should put on your own oxygen mask before helping others. If you get too weak from lack of oxygen, you'll be of no use to the other person. Similarly, if a physician's well-being isn't taken care of, the physician will be of no use to the patient. The physician needs to be taught to put on their own oxygen mask first before helping the patient. Not the other way around.

Unfortunately, this isn't the case. As a result, physicians work themselves to the bone and don't take time to adequately recover. This is disastrous. Last time I checked, physicians were humans, not superheroes with infinite energy supplies. So, until physicians become Captain Americas, the mantra should be "the physician's well-being always comes first, so that the physician can help the patient be healthy."

When I was finishing up residency, work-hour schedule limitation rules came into effect. However, many residents stayed beyond the allocated time to complete all the tasks required to take care of patients (paperwork, checking labs, etc.). In addition, being able to stay beyond the required work hours and function efficiently was considered a badge of honour. Fast-forward to attendinghood. Some physicians continue to ignore their physical and emotional health. Not only does this affect the physician's ability to deliver good care to the patient, but it can also affect the patient's ability to listen to the physician's advice. For example, a cardiologist who is significantly obese won't be taken as seriously by a patient when it comes to diet modification. Physicians, just like everyone else, are judged on appearance.

Since physicians tend to lack balance in regards to taking care of themselves, they may be more prone to react poorly to other stresses in life. For example, an elderly parent becoming ill is stressful for any child. But a physician may not be able to cope effectively with this situation if the well is already dry from lack of self-care.

6. THE BURNOUT CURE

WHAT DO we do about burnout, institutionally and individually?

When You're Burned Out

If you're a burned out physician, perhaps you're thinking about changing jobs. Maybe switching from a hospital-employed position to an outpatient-concierge position is the answer? In some cases, switching your location or job type may indeed be the answer. If so, that's wonderful.

Switching jobs may seem great in the short term, during the honeymoon period, but not likely in the long term. Unfortunately, if you're in the healthcare industry, certain environmental factors will follow you no matter where you go or what job you hold. Working in medicine is always going to be stressful—we're taking care of people's health. Working in medicine is always going to involve personality conflicts because we're working with people—patients and office staff.

It's also hard to predict what a job will be like before you start, as people tend to put their best sides forward during interviews. Do your research before determining that changing jobs is really the answer, because doing so isn't an easy task, at least in the United States.

To change jobs in the US, a physician is often required to give three months' notice. Also, individual states have laws on patient abandonment, so that patient care is transferred adequately. And most medical contracts have noncompete clauses that stipulate a physician cannot practice nearby for at least a year or more. For a physician, leaving a job can mean physically relocating. If this relocation is to a new state, they may have to wait a few months to get a new state license. Once credentialed in a new state, they need to get credentialed by insurance companies and hospitals. Not to mention they'll need to transfer things such as Medicare numbers, Medicaid numbers, and DEA licenses to their new location of practice. Finally, when a physician leaves a medical practice, they often have to pay something called tail insurance. This way, after they leave, they'll still have malpractice coverage if someone sues them. Since the United States is a litigious society, getting tail insurance is a no-brainer. But this insurance can cost tens of thousands of dollars, depending on the state and specialty.

Institutional Change

To address physician burnout, the institutions—from medical schools to hospitals and medical licensing boards—need to change. We are slowly starting to see change at an institutional level. In June 2017, it was announced that Dr. Tait Shanafelt would become the chief wellness officer at Stanford Medical School. This was the first such hire for a US academic medical center.[1] Then, in October 2017, the first American Conference on Physician Health was held in San Francisco.[2] The conference was cosponsored by the American Medical Association and the Mayo Clinic, in conjunction with Stanford. Hopefully, we'll see many more institutional-level changes like these in the future.

There are also wonderful grassroots changes happening. Dr.

Dike Drummond is a physician burnout expert who runs a site called the Happy MD.[3]

Even one of my old medical school colleagues has gotten in on the action. Dr. Michael Lee has always had a strong interest in physician health. In an interview with Thomas Yoon, he discusses the topic of empathy with boundaries.[4]

This is a very important concept for physicians. It's fine for a physician to have empathy, of course, but we need boundaries to hold patients and staff members accountable for their actions. For example, if a patient uses more medication than prescribed because of a stressful life event, the physician can empathize with the patient but the patient should still be held accountable for their actions and be restricted on future prescriptions.

While the issue of physician burnout is a serious one today, I see hope on the horizon. The community is starting to acknowledge that the healer needs healing.

My generation may not see a complete change in the system, but hopefully it will only continue to improve for those who come afterward. I hope to contribute to the solution by sharing the lessons I learned through comedy.

MY COMEDIC ADVENTURES

SECTION TWO

7. THE FLAME CHALLENGE

I'D SWITCHED to a self-employed position in early 2013 and had increased the duration of my patient appointment slots, but I still felt like medicine was an assembly line prison.

A recurring theme was my inability to communicate. On one hand, friends who weren't doctors often told me about their frustration with the lack of time available to ask questions of their physicians. Other physicians and I often discussed our frustration with the lack of time available to connect with patients.

It was this frustration that drove me to want to learn how to communicate better to patients—in the hopes it would help make my job somewhat tolerable. That meant undoing much of what I'd been trained and conditioned to do during medical school, where we were taught the *medical way* to communicate.

I had no idea that this would lead me into the multiple flavors of comedy, or that the challenge of going so far out of my comfort zone would reinvigorate my inner flame. The change of perspective would heal the healer.

It started out with a writing competition designed to communicate science to non-scientists. A fellow physician told me about a competition called The Flame Challenge[1], in which scientists answered a question by way of a short written or video entry. She suggested I enter the competition as a way to learn more about effective communication. The panel of judges was the coolest thing about the competition—eleven- and twelve-year-old children from around the world.

The Flame Challenge

The Flame Challenge came into existence through the work of Alan Alda[2], an actor famous for playing Hawkeye, a sarcastic, realistic, caring physician on M*A*S*H. M*A*S*H was a television sitcom that featured a medical unit in a war zone during the Korean War. Alda went on to host the show *Scientific American Frontiers*. When Alda was a child, he asked a teacher, "What is a flame?" The teacher's response was so complex and full of jargon, Alda couldn't understand it. The premise of The Flame Challenge was that if a scientist could make a child understand a scientific concept that was a communication success.[3]

In 2015, The Flame Challenge question was "What is sleep?" This seemed like the perfect question for me to answer, since sleep was my subspecialty. Day in and day out, I answered questions regarding sleep in my clinic. However, this didn't mean it was easy for me to answer the question for the competition.

1. The written entries had to be under 250 words. Given that I knew a lot about the subject, it was hard to determine what to include. It was even harder to decide what to leave out.
2. The question was expansive and open-ended. I was used to answering pointed questions regarding specific conditions or testing results.
3. I was acutely aware that I was writing for children. How was I going to capture the attention of a child?

My solution? Dolphins.
Here's my entry:

Did you know a bottle-nose dolphin's brain can be asleep and awake at the same time? While one half of the brain sleeps, the other half stays awake!
When humans go to sleep at night, our whole brain and body goes to sleep all at once.
Whether you are a dolphin or a human, we both need sleep to survive. Sleep is your daily, rest mini-vacation for both the brain and the body. Sleep gives you a break so that you can get ready for the next day.
When you are asleep, you go back and forth between REM and non-REM sleep every 90 minutes. That is about four to five times a night.
REM stands for rapid eye movement. During REM sleep, even though your eyes move back and forth rapidly under your eyelids, the rest of body's muscles are completely relaxed. Your heart beats faster and your breathing is not as regular. This is also the part of sleep during which you remember your dreams. During REM sleep, your brain's energy is restored. Good REM sleep helps you get good grades.
During non-REM sleep, breathing slows down and blood supply increases to the muscles. During non-REM sleep, hormones such as growth hormone are released. These hormones are essential for growth and repair of muscle tissue. During non-REM sleep, you body's muscle energy is restored. Good non-REM sleep helps you run really fast.
But, sleep is not just important for grades and running. When you don't sleep well, you get sick, feel cranky and fall asleep during your favorite movie!
How much sleep do you need? Dolphins sleep about eight hours a

day. Most ten- to twelve-year-olds need nine to eleven hours a day. So, make sure you get more sleep than a dolphin!

IN THE SPRING OF 2015, I was notified that my entry was one of the three finalists in the written category of The Flame Challenge. After the finalists were announced, Alan Alda interviewed a few of the children reviewing the entries. Discussing my entry, one young lady remarked that she liked the dolphin aspect but that the middle of the entry was pretty boring. I reread my entry with her comments in mind and found she was right. The beginning and ending were strong, but the middle was definitely not up to snuff!

The Flame Challenge Applied

Did I win the competition? Nope. But the process taught me quite a bit about communicating science to the non-scientific community.

I learned the importance of not using overly technical language. When a physician slips into doctor speak with patients, it becomes harder for the patient to understand what the physician is trying to tell them.

The 250-word limit of the entry helped me learn to be concise. This is also a very good skill to have as a physician. Patients can digest only a small amount of information at one time, especially if the subject is new to them. The importance of brevity is further compounded by ever-shortening appointment times.

And I learned that if information isn't presented in an engaging way, the patient's attention may wander. All in all, if the physician doesn't communicate properly, they can come off looking robotic and uncaring.

After the Challenge

The Flame Challenge wasn't just a great learning experience—it was also my first chance in a long time to do something creative. One Sunday afternoon after the challenge, I found a quiet location in my apartment, grabbed a pen and a piece of paper, and set a timer for fifteen minutes. I purposely turned the timer around so I couldn't see the numbers. Then I wrote down as quickly as I could everything that I'd enjoyed prior to medical school. I didn't think. I just wrote. Afterward, it took me quite a while to decipher what I'd written. Most people know that physicians are notorious for having bad handwriting. Well, in medical school, my professors used to joke that my handwriting was so bad it could be used as an example for other medical students of how not to write.

After reviewing my list, I circled the three things I'd enjoyed the most: art-museum visits, dance, and music. Before attending medical school, I frequented art museums quite a bit. Sitting among paintings gave me a sense of peace. In terms of dance, during high school, I performed an Indian classical dance called Kuchipudi. After high school, I didn't perform on a regular basis but enjoyed simply dancing around the living room. It gave me a sense of joy. And prior to attending medical school, I frequented an area of Washington, DC, called Adams Morgan. Back in those days, it was somewhat rundown and had little-known cafes and clubs. I loved to show up solo to intimate venues, sit in the back, and just take in the musicians. It gave me a sense of wonderment.

I looked again at my top three items and recircled music. Then I laid out a plan to bring music back into my life. Given that I was in my late thirties, going out to clubs late at night, as I'd done in my early twenties, seemed a far stretch. My tolerance for smoke fumes and raucous drunkards had decreased significantly. So I decided to listen to more music. For a few months, I made it a point to listen to music for at least fifteen minutes a day, and it became a habit. I rediscovered that long lost sense of wonderment.

This exercise didn't seem important at the time, but it ended up being a key prelude to my comedy journey. Comedy requires one to let go, get uncomfortable, and be vulnerable. Reconnecting with part of my pre-medical school persona was the first step in this journey.

After The Flame Challenge ended, I did more research on Alan Alda and learned that he taught improv classes to scientists. That piqued my interest, and led to the second step on my comedy journey.

I Googled "improvisation lessons." The first item that came up was a multi-week level one course at the DC Improv. Like The Flame Challenge, I figured it would be a good exercise in communication. With a series of clicks and a hard swallow, I signed up.

8. ZIP ZAP ZOP

ON A WARM SUNDAY morning in September, notebook in hand, I boarded a bus and headed off to Dupont Circle, a popular neighborhood with great dining and nightlife in Washington, DC. I'd been to Dupont thousands of times over the course of my tenure in the Washington area, yet I couldn't recall having seen a place called DC Improv.

I ended up at a set of stairs leading down to a basement comedy club.

I hadn't realized that I was signing up for *comedy* improvisation classes. In fact, I didn't know there were different kinds of improv. I knew even less about comedy. Sure, I'd seen sitcoms on television. But I was a complete novice when it came to the history of comedy. I didn't know, for example, that DC Improv had been hosting big names in comedy for more than twenty years. I'd simply chosen classes at this location because it was easy to get to and at the top of a Google-search list.

I had envisioned a class in which we'd all sit around in a circle discussing techniques and then we'd do some homework. I'd expected a time commitment of only few hours on a Sunday for a couple of weeks. *What's the harm?* I thought.

Down the stairs I went, and a nice person sitting in a ticket-taking area directed me into a smaller room to the left. I would later find out that this was the venue for the more intimate shows. There was a small stage at the front and a big clearing in the middle of the room with chairs and circular tables pushed out to the edges. Pictures of apparently famous people plastered the wall. The only one I recognized was Seinfeld. I had only watched *Saturday Night Live* maybe once or twice in my life.

Some of the students in this class were actors or comedians who wanted to learn comedy for their careers. Some were professionals looking for a way to let off steam—there were quite a few management consultants in this class. As a sleep specialist, I treated many management consultants for insomnia issues, so I wasn't surprised they needed to release some stress. But everyone in the class seemed to know something about comedy. I knew nothing.

The club owner, a lovely curly-haired gal, welcomed us to the club. She introduced herself and the instructor. He asked everybody to introduce themselves.

With that out of the way, I opened my notebook, ready to listen to some theory for the next few hours. Instead, the instructor told us to get up, move to the center of the room, and form a circle. We were to start playing a game.

What? No precise instructions, no demonstrations, no handouts? We were just supposed to improvise?

My mind was churning like a ferris wheel at the prospect of being spontaneous in front of a group of complete strangers. Thanks to my medical training, I kept a calm demeanor. But inside I was panicking.

The Physician Machine

Let's roll the camera back from this scene for a minute.

You have to understand that medical training helps to program we physicians into algorithmic creatures. When a patient presents with X, Y, and Z, you go down different nodes of a decision-making tree depending on the information received. This training is important. Physicians must quickly and easily decide on the right diagnostic and treatment pathways. If you were a patient who'd just arrived in an emergency room, you wouldn't want your physician to sit there, tapping her toes, while deliberating about whether to start you on a nebulizer breathing treatment or administer an aspirin.

These algorithmic medical decision-making trees contribute to making physicians cautious. As we should be.

However, the negative side of this training is that sometimes we can seem so mechanical that we don't connect with our patients on a human level.

The first rule of medicine is "do no harm." Given that I was naturally serious before I became a doctor, medicine made me even more cautious. I would say I'd become extremely cautious. Especially since I was practicing in the litigious United States, where there are a lot of medical lawsuits.

So, you can perhaps understand the complete and utter fear I felt when I had to get up and improvise in front of this group.

Back to the Basement

How was I going to manage to play a silly game with these strangers? In fact, how was I going to do comedy? I was about as funny as a dull doorknob.

That first game involved passing an imaginary ball around to help us remember each other's names. This wasn't too bad. Next came a game where the first person was to say "zip" and point to another person around the circle. The person pointed to immediately pointed at someone else and said "zap." The third person repeated the pointing gesture and said, "zop." On and on this went, faster and faster, becoming harder and harder to keep track of who was being pointed at and what their next word in the sequence was.

Each new game got progressively more vexing. The last game of that first day was the worst by far. People stood around you in a circle while you sang with all the power in your lungs. For me, improvising was bad enough—singing in public was even worse. The only thing my singing is good for is to get dogs barking. Seriously, how much more embarrassing could this day get?

If my medical training helped me put up a calm outward appearance regardless how I felt inside, people who don't know me well might wonder if I have a pulse. I'm not prone to emotional outbursts or violence. But when I was told to sing while standing in a circle of strangers, I thought I might explode.

When that first class was done, I burst out of the room as fast as I could, in that moment telling myself there was no way I was going back to that nutter house.

If I hadn't paid in full in advance for the entire class, I would never have gone back. But I had, and so I did. Go back, that is. Week after week. Plus, there was something inside of me that wanted to conquer the challenge—we medical folk can be quite determined. After all, I had survived medical school. Surely I could survive an improvisation class.

The management consultants in the course seemed at least as embarrassed as I was and that helped me feel more at ease. I was still horrible at improv. But to my surprise, I found that it was like play for adults and I was actually enjoying myself. Just a little.

A few of my classmates shared that they were moving on to level two, which was a performance class. I figured performing a pretend show in front of the class on the small stage was something I could do, so I decided to sign up.

Level two classes were held on Thursday nights rather than Sundays. Coming from the clinic, I was in doctor mode and it was much harder for me to get into the improv mode. To my horror, I learned that the performance show would be held in the big comedy room which seated a few hundred people.

This performance class pushed me further beyond my comfort zone than I had been in a long time. Which had tremendous value for me, because by this point I hated medicine so much that going back to my previous state of existence was no longer an option.

9. THE CONNECTION CONUNDRUM

ON DECEMBER 8TH, 2015, I ended up performing—really, really badly. And you know what? It didn't kill me.

I felt tremendous pressure to be funny. But consider the words of Mick Napier, improv theater teacher: "Some of the best scenes I've ever seen are those that are about not getting laughs."[1]

I learned that improvisation isn't really about making people laugh—it's about human connection in the present moment. And this ability to connect in the here and now can be of great benefit to physicians wishing to connect with patients in the clinical office.

Physicians, already trained in their machine-like processing of diagnostic decision trees, are further challenged when trying to read beyond what a patient might be saying. Patients are often very good at hiding how they're really feeling.

In his book on relating and communicating, Alan Alda describes research that examined whether physicians and patients were in sync during therapy sessions. The study involved reviewing video-taped sessions and measuring parameters such as skin conductance. The findings concluded a significant emotional gap exists between patient and doctor, as patients can outwardly hide their emotions.[2]

In clinical practice, as a regular physician I didn't have the time or resources to measure and review patients in this way. I'm a physician, not a body language expert. However, by learning some basic improvisation techniques, I found I could better listen to my patients' words, tone, and body language. Improvisation allowed me as the physician to become more creative and to connect beyond my algorithmic programming. It was all about flexing what I call the present-tense muscles.

Present Tense Muscles

Present tense muscles allow the physician to bridge the connection gap between doctor and patient in the present moment. I discovered five ways that improv really helped me to strengthen my present-tense muscles.

1. Listening

In improv, there are many games in which you need to really listen to what other people are saying. As Stephen Covey noted in *The 7 Habits of Highly Effective People*, "Most people do not listen with the intent to understand; they listen with the intent to reply."[3]

When a patient is speaking, instead of really listening, the physician is going down the decision-making tree to determine what tests to order and what treatments are needed. Unfortunately, when the physician isn't really listening, we miss important clues in a patient's history.

One listening-training game I played in my comedy improv class is called Dr. No. In this game, a group of people line up on stage. The audience asks a question, and the people on stage must answer. However, each person in the group can only say one word at a time to form the reply. For example, if the question is, "What is the weather like?" the first person in the line says, "the," the second person says, "weather," the third person says, "is," and so forth. This game helped teach me to listen closely to everybody's individual words instead of the gist of the sentence as a whole.

2. Observing

Other improv games require you to observe the gestures, postures, and other body language closely. We played a movement game that involves standing in a circle and throwing a pretend ball. After the ball has been passed around for a while, a second item, such as a knife, is introduced. Catching each pretend object requires a different gesture. You'd catch the ball with two open hands. You'd catch the knife by closing one or both hands around the handle. By closely observing the movements of the others in the circle, I became much better at being ready for the objects heading in my direction.

3. Mirroring

Mirroring works like this: if your partner lifts his left arm, you lift your right arm. If your partner smiles with the left side of his mouth, so do you on the right side of your face. The advantage of mirror training is that it helps partners to be really in sync with each other during a conversation.

Mirroring people, their language and gestures, often makes them feel more comfortable. It also allows for better connection with partners in improv, and it can also make for better connection between doctor and patient in the medical treatment room.

4. Tone

Much of what's communicated verbally is through tone rather than the choice of words. In a game called Alien, one player is the interpreter and the other player is the alien. The interpreter must come up with a translation for the audience of the alien's foreign language, based solely on their gestures and tone.

5. Listening and Observing

The next layer of communicative understanding involves putting the listening and observing together at the same time. Here's the simple exercise we used to practice this. Standing in a circle once again, one person would create a sound and physical motion. The person next to them would receive the sound and motion and react in a way that feels natural. Person three, reacts, interprets, and passes onto the next, and so on. By the time each person in the circle has interacted with the sound and physical motion, both will have changed quite a bit. The point of this exercise isn't to attempt to preserve and replicate the original sound and motion, but to feel their intent and use that to generate your own sound and movement. This exercise can train physicians to pay attention to patients' physical language and tone instead of just their words, and also to react to those cues.

2016 Forward

When I finished my performance class, in December 2015, I thought I was done with comedy improvisation. I had accomplished my goal of learning a few new communication tools and venturing well outside of my comfort zone. In early 2016 I would be traveling to South America—I was not considering a continuation of comedic improv.

Fast forward to spring 2016. I was in yet another comedy improv class. Intellectually, I told myself it was to learn more communication skills. Emotionally, I loved the playful release of improv. For the next two years, I took more improv classes, went to improv group meet-ups, and learned many lessons to aid me in the medical office.

I also discovered that improv helped me get out of my loner shell. Improv is about, "Yes, and," not, "Yes, but." Performers have to work with each other, not get in the way of each other. If your improv partner starts a scene by walking through a shoe shop, you could become the salesperson, another customer, or even a shoe. These choices mean you're saying, "Yes, and," to your partner. However, if your partner starts a scene about walking through a shoe shop and you say that the shoe store burned down, that would be saying, "Yes, but." Instead of honoring your scene partner's choice, you would be making a choice that conflicts with it. "Yes, and," showed me a way to stop working as though I were alone in a perfectionist manner and start working in a more cooperative one.

Improvisation increases contextual awareness. Because you have to pay attention to everything about your scene partner—tone, voice, physicality, gestures, story, and more—context is important. Your partner may be talking about getting lost and asking for directions, but your response will be different depending on the context of the scene. Is your partner asking for directions in a shopping mall or remote village surrounded by thick forest? Is your partner acting nervous or confident? Each scenario will evoke a different reaction. Context is everything in improv.

Paying attention to context in improv not only helped me pay attention to patients, coworkers, and loved ones, but also to myself. Improv gave me an increased sense of self-awareness.

For physicians who have become burned out, self-awareness is highly beneficial. Being honest with themselves about what it is about medicine they do and don't like can make a big difference on the road to recovery.

Improv increased my self-awareness to the point where I realized how much I disliked medicine. When I started as an attending physician, I thought my discomfort stemmed from little things I could change, such as appointment times or paperwork overload. When I added all the little things up, I found that my frustration was enormous. Improv helped me understand that my dislike was nourished by much deeper roots.

To this day, I'm still horrible at comedy improv. But instead of wanting to run away, I love taking part when I have the chance. Call me an improv convert.

I feel welcome in the comedy improv community. It's a diverse group of people who come together to form spontaneous scenes. Improv is a form of play. Improv doesn't just spark laughter—it fosters spontaneous creativity. A random scene from improvisation often sparked the start of a short story or reminded me of a dance. This creativity overflowed into many areas of my life. One of the greatest gifts my improv classes gave me was the people.

10. FOREIGN ACCENTS

EVERY TIME I stepped on the stage to perform a scene in my improv classes, I felt butterflies in my stomach. But I'd learned to befriend the fear. I took comfort in being on stage with others.

A few people from my improv classes signed up for the stand-up comedy class at the DC Improv. The idea of being on the stage by myself seemed terrifying. On the other hand, the material was prepared instead of spontaneous. I reasoned that the ability to prepare my material in advance would offset the fear of being alone on stage. The world of stand-up would open up yet another new world of communication.

My Sociology Education

I took a stand-up comedy class in the fall of 2016 and another in the spring of 2017. The classes provided some excellent techniques, but the real learning came from performing at local comedy shows.

Restaurants and bars hosted open mic nights, during which comics could perform in front of patrons. The more experienced comics got their slots earlier in the evening, while those of us who were inexperienced would get up on stage toward the end of the lineup. To perform at these open mics, it wasn't unusual to have to wait around until after 11:00 p.m. or even midnight. And the shows were on weeknights, with the weekend shows saved for the pros.

By the time I was trying my hand at open mics, I was on the cusp of turning forty. My idea of a late night was staying out past 8:00 p.m. If people asked me to dinner, I'd suggest brunch. So, hauling myself to open mics, especially on weeknights, I might have been up for this in my twenties, but not anymore. At the bars, while waiting for my turn to perform, I'd ask for decaffeinated tea with milk instead of a drink. When they didn't have decaf tea, I'd settle for a soft drink or water.

Pre-standup, given my profession and Indian heritage, my usual network sphere of acquaintances tended toward the upper class of people with at least one graduate degree. In the world of stand-up, I was exposed to a very different demographic. Stand-up attracted a mixed crowd.

There were the twentysomethings just starting out and older comics who'd been at it for a while and really loved the craft. During their routines, the comics often made fun of experiences from their everyday lives. To me, it was like a sociological investigation. I got to hear about wide-ranging experiences from ethnic and economic worlds to which I'd never been exposed outside the confines of my medical practice. It gave me a greater appreciation for the hardships people faced. The stand-up routines weren't just about humor—they also provided social commentary. Did I always agree with the opinions? No. But I was open to hearing them.

Most comics don't get rich or famous. They have day jobs and do comedy after hours. Some of the most dedicated comics I met went to open mics four or five nights a week, and sometimes to two or three open mics in one night. They knew that the best way to hone their craft was repetition, repetition, and more repetition.

I admired their tenacity. It wasn't easy to get up there in front of audiences, especially those who gave only muted applause.

Many open mic night comics recorded their performances so they could later review which parts had gotten laughs and which parts were weak. They'd use the feedback to adjust their words, tone, pace, gestures, and expressions to deliver a better effect. The good comics could also read the audience in real time and make adjustments on the fly. A Wednesday-night-after-work crowd is very different from a late-Saturday-night crowd. I was amazed by how one comic could take one line and rework it over and over again in order to connect with the audience more effectively. The goal wasn't just to make people laugh, but also to connect with the audience and make a lasting impression.

Parana, Pepperoni, Pikachu, and Premise

As the comic Haywood Turnipseed Jr. told me, a great comedy act is like a great melody—it's all about timing.[1] Watching seasoned comics perform is like watching a seasoned musician: they time their beats perfectly.

A stand-up comedian's set (aka performance) is built around premises. Through these premises, they connect with the audience. For example, one premise in my set is the fact that people have come up with many versions of my name over the years. In general, stand-up comics follow the rule of threes—they create three jokes around a premise, the last one often the most powerful. Another way to use this rule is to tell two jokes that are expected and a third with an unexpected twist. The opening line of my set was something to the effect of, "My name is Pranathi. Not Parana, Miss Pepperoni, or, as my neighbor's kid likes to call me, Miss Pikachu." (On paper, the joke doesn't have quite the same effect.) Originally, I had different versions of the mispronunciations of my name. Trying them out on different audiences and observing the responses, I was able to optimize the mispronunciation choices and their order. I also added character voices to heighten the effect.

Stand-up can also involve taking something that is known and exaggerating it for effect. For example, in medicine, physicians constantly face ludicrous policies, imposed by administrators, that aren't beneficial to patients. So in one line of my set, I mocked an administrator trying to save money.

Administrator: "You now have one-and-a-half patient slots."

Doctor: "So, if a patient shows up for a half patient slot and has a weak left hand and a twitch in his right hand, well, I'll have to tell Mr. Klaus, 'I'm sorry, you're in the half patient slot, so you've got to pick. Weakness or twitch. Can't do both.'"

Brevity and timing are also key. Stand-up comics are known for packing a punch with as few words as possible. Every word is carefully chosen and has a specific purpose. If it doesn't work, it's taken out.

The Clinical Time Crunch

This stand-up comedy notion of getting your message across effectively in the smallest amount of time comes in handy during short clinical office visits. Stand-up requires assessing an audience's response to your routine in real time, so you can adjust your delivery. As a physician, being able to read your patients and adjust your message based on their reactions is a very important skill.

In the US medical system in 2018, an average return-patient visit was fifteen minutes. This fifteen minutes translates into five to ten minutes of real conversation. Most new-patient appointments are thirty to forty-five minutes, which translates into twenty to thirty minutes of real conversation. Ironically, I often feel as though I need more time with a return patient than a new one because there are often tests to review. As a sleep specialist, I'm somewhat lucky in that my concentrated time frame can be focused on one clinical arena. I really feel for primary care physicians who have to cover many more topics in a concentrated time period.

Another challenge that presents itself during short office visits is the distance that vulnerability creates between patient and physician. Many patients often feel nervous and vulnerable entering a clinical encounter in which they must discuss personal details. Many physicians, even if they don't mean to, can come across as arrogant because they focus on the medical aspect of the visit instead of the human one. Of course, the patient is visiting for medical treatment, but if the physician doesn't take time to acknowledge the human side of the issue, the patient can feel like a number instead of a human being, decreasing both the feeling of connection and their willingness to follow through on the medical advice.

If physicians can once in a while feel raw vulnerability and utter exposure (it doesn't necessarily have to involve comedy), they will find themselves reminded of what patients often go through in medical settings. And a reminder of patients' realities can remind us to make the human connection, no matter how short the clinical visit time.

Trying my hand at open mic stand-up comedy helped me bridge this distance and vulnerability gap. Feeling completely exposed increased my empathy with patients. It took a great deal of guts. And a good cup of tea didn't hurt.

Humorous Honesty Heals

I became bitter working in clinical medicine. It seemed I'd spent years on training only to work in a machine-like job in which billing was more important than healing. Taking my issues within medicine and translating them into a stand-up routine was cathartic. While things such as mispronunciations of my name, ludicrous administration demands, and insurance company ridiculousness were easy to make fun of, the topic that was harder to broach was my mistreatment by patients.

I had a few patients saying and doing things that were completely inappropriate. I had a patient who asked me whether I was from Detroit, Michigan or Detroit, Iran. When I told him I went to high school in Detroit, Michigan, he breathed a sigh of relief. He explained that if I were from Iran, the CPAP machine could be a bomb. I'm not sure why the patient thought he was important enough to warrant my coming over as a special agent from Iran just to bomb him.

When I complained to my superiors, I was told to keep quiet—we couldn't displease the patient because the patient is the customer. Over the years, I grew firmer in my demands to have inappropriate patients reassigned, which angered my administrators. Most of the patients who were overtly sexually inappropriate were reassigned. However, the racist ones weren't. I had to try to treat them and move on.

Incorporating some of these ridiculous incidents into my stand-up routine proved to be an effective outlet.

In going to and performing in these open mics and listening to comics online, I came to admire the comics who were able to raise issues of concern through humor. When a serious topic is presented with humor, it's often better received. Humor can soften the delivery. The more I studied stand-up, the more I realized that the truth provided the best comedy and had the ability to heal. Whether it be humor about what really happens in the physician's office or humor about what happens as a first-time parent, great stand-up comedy has the ability to highlight other people's everyday realities, of which the audience is otherwise unaware.

Before I leave the topic of honesty: at open mic comedy nights, I never told anybody that I was a physician. If someone asked me what I did, I didn't lie. But I didn't volunteer this information. People tend to have a load of preconceived notions about doctors.

They may treat you differently. They may try to get medical advice. They may not feel comfortable talking around you. They may assume you're more intelligent, more obnoxious, or rich—some people have even hit me up for money. In my experience, when I tell people I'm a physician, it creates a distance and not in a good way. It was important to me to go to these open mics and interact with other comics and the audience on an even plane. A great deal of my routine was about medicine, of course. But the important thing is that I didn't want special treatment before getting on stage. I wanted to feel the same vulnerability as other comics.

The Dark Side

Comedy can sometimes push boundaries, and buttons, and unfortunately some comic routines are downright inappropriate. I've been appalled at some jokes or entire routines, surprised at the raucous applause. I believe that sweeping generalizations that mock entire groups of people, no matter who they are, are inappropriate.

Comics who play to generalities get the low-hanging laughs. But those who point out social issues by taking the high road instead of the low road are, in my humble opinion, the true giants of the craft. Great comedy doesn't stoop down but enlightens and lifts up. If you decide to take up stand-up, choose to be a giant!

And remember, it doesn't matter whether you're a man or a woman, black or white, gay or straight, old or young, rich or poor, native or foreign, have disabilities or don't, love thin-crust pizza or thick-crust pizza—laughter has no foreign accent.

11. EDUCATE, ENTERTAIN, INSPIRE

BETWEEN 2015 AND 2017, my life was filled with comedic improv and stand-up adventures, but eventually, real life kicked in. I couldn't get through the late open mics very well, even if I substituted full-strength coffee for my decaf tea. As a more mature creature, I'd gotten to the point where I'd rather be home curled up with a favorite movie than out at a bar.

I continued to partake in informal comedy improv jams whenever I got the chance. They're a great way for me to spark creativity. But I wanted a different outlet for comedy—one that didn't require stage time. And so, in the winter of 2017, I took a sketch comedy writing class, and in the fall of 2017, I took a workshop in satire writing.

Now, I won't pretend a class here and there makes one proficient in comedy writing. But these classes did open my eyes to the power of the written word in spreading important messages.

The Janitor

Before I took these writing classes, my main exposure to comedic writing was through television shows. Growing up in England, I'd watched classics such as *'Allo 'Allo!* and *Yes, Prime Minister*. After moving to America, I regularly watched *Friends, The Fresh Prince of Bel-Air*, and *Frasier*. And in 2001, during my internship year (my first year after medical school), an American comedy series called *Scrubs* aired. This show was a humorous look at the adventures of a group of interns.

As the interns on *Scrubs* matured in their respective careers, I matured in mine. Even though the issues the characters faced are portrayed in a humorous context, *Scrubs* is still one of the most realistic shows I've seen in terms of the portrayal of medicine and the issues that physicians face.

These days, when you ask a person to name a medical show, they might say *Grey's Anatomy*. I admire Shonda Rhimes's writing immensely. I also appreciate the perfect description of workplace burnout she described in her TED talk: "When your job tastes like dust."[1] But the lives of actual physicians are quite different from how they're portrayed on *Grey's Anatomy*. I only wish most surgeons had the body of McSteamy.

Other medical shows showcase specific components of medicine quite well. *House* includes wonderful details regarding medical diagnoses. I loved watching Hugh Laurie brilliantly portray an investigator who cured obscure medical conditions. For fifteen years, *ER* showcased a Chicago emergency room with eye-opening artistry. *M*A*S*H* beautifully illustrated the realities of war-time medicine on the frontlines.

While all these shows highlight important facets of medicine, none of them quite takes viewers inside the psyche of a physician the way *Scrubs* does. In *Scrubs*, most scenes take place through the eyes of the main character, Dr. John Dorian, aka J.D. Each episode starts and ends with his narration. His funny daydreams feature prominently. They're funny but they also provide an important look at the inner dialogue of a physician.[2]

The series delves into the interns' relationships with other hospital staff, such as nurses, senior residents, and senior medical staff. One of the funniest relationships is between the janitor and J.D. The janitor doesn't seem to like J.D. and always causes trouble for him at work. Most physicians can relate. My so-called janitor was a ward clerk during my neurology residency. Whenever we worked a shift together, she always questioned my orders and never acted on them without substantial effort on my part. Ironically, when it came time for me to leave, she gave me a cake and cried over my departure.

Doctor and Patient Dating

The outcome of my writing classes was a sketch in which a patient goes to a speed-dating-to-find-a-doctor night. She "dates" several different physicians: an obnoxious know-it-all, a hippie feelgooder, a non-responder, one who's fixated on his computer screen, and another who only pays attention to his stocks. At the end of the sketch, she ends up choosing the waitress as her physician. Granted, this scenario isn't realistic, and the physician stereotypes were exaggerated. However, the characters I presented in my sketch grew out of actual patient complaints I've heard.

I also wrote a sketch in which a doctor goes to a restaurant to meet the perfect patient. The doctor meets an obnoxious know-it-all, an alternative-medicine addict, a non-responder, one who's fixated on his cell phone, and one who's passive aggressive. At the end of the sketch, the doctor decides to quit medicine and become a waitress to get more respect. Again, this scenario isn't realistic and the patient stereotypes were exaggerations. But these characters were based on real live patients I've had in my practice.

My sketches will never see the light of day on any stage and are meant for my own comedic release. But luckily, many physicians who do have a talent for writing satire are taking their work further than their own desks.

Satire is often topical and uses humor, irony, and exaggeration to illustrate or make fun of shortcomings. A good example is a piece in which the merits of a sweet potato are overblown. Comedy writer Caitlin Kunkel notes that she ate a sweet potato and "overnight, [she] became a paragon of fitness and health inspiration for those around [her]."[3] Now, consider all the health supplements and revolutionary medical treatments that promise life-changing results being advertised on TV and online. Hyperbole is everywhere within the health-and-wellness consumer space. Medicine is indeed ripe for satire.

Entertain. Educate. Inspire.

On an episode of *The Creative Penn*, a podcast for writers, the host says, "People don't buy books. They buy entertainment, inspiration, or information."[4] The same applies to videos. Comedic videos about medicine entertain, educate, and inspire all at the same time.

My medical training took place long before the age of YouTube. Even if I were training today, I don't think I'd have the nerve to sing and dance for a video and stick it up on YouTube. But if you search "medical parody videos," you'll find medical students doing parodies of everything from Disney-movie songs to dance sequences. For example, "First Year Funk" is a parody of Bruno Mars's "Uptown Funk." The lyrics are changed to reflect the travail of being a first-year medical student.[5] And in "Let Me Go," a student parodies the Disney song "Let It Go" to depict the hardships of a third-year medical student's clinical rotations.[6]

In this age of medical parodies, one physician stands out. Remember Dr. Zubin Damania and his alter-ego ZDoggMD that I mentioned in section one? He's been making musical parodies on a variety of medical topics. Some focus on educating patients. In one he has a song about how to recognize if somebody is having a stroke.[7] His major appeal lies in his ability to depict the reality of the field. For example, in "EHR State of Mind," he educates the public on the ridiculousness of electronic medical records.[8] Originally, he started making videos as a release for his burnout. Now, he has a large online following looking to be entertained, educated, and, more importantly, inspired to action.

While comedic writing can't solve all the problems in our healthcare system, it can start to make a positive dent in it and is a powerful tool for change.

THE COMEDIC CURE

SECTION THREE

12. THE GOOD OF A SIMPLE SMILE

AT ITS CORE, comedy is about connecting with the audience. Whether it's an improv scene about baking pumpkin pies, a written sketch about doctor dating, or a stand-up performance of a joke about hospital administration, it's a chance to make a real connection.

In a similar way, every time a physician sees a patient, they have a chance to make a real connection.

Connections like these are about communication, and communication based on what I've learned from comedy can be broken into three major themes: story, presence, and engagement.

Story

A story recounts events or people for the purposes of entertainment, information, or inspiration.

The words of authors who've been dead for hundreds of years continue to resonate around the world. This is because stories carry the fabric of our culture. Regardless of our race, religion, sex, or socioeconomic status, we all have stories we can relate to. While I'm drawn to fantasy, romance, historical fiction, and maybe a splash of science fiction, all the books that really resonate with me have a degree of good conquering evil, an element of a love story, and sprinkles of intelligent humor. Pure mystery and horror stories don't hold much appeal for me—not because these genres are any less valuable but because different stories resonate with different souls. No matter what type of story you enjoy, it's hard to argue against the universal appeal of story. They span centuries and cultures.

Why is the value of story so universal? Part of the reason is neurobiology. The human brain looks like a mushroom with a stalk. It's made up of three parts: the brainstem, or stalk, is the most ancient part of the brain (from an evolutionary standpoint) and is responsible for vital functions like breathing and heart rate control. The middle or limbic part of the brain is the emotional center. The head of the mushroom is home to higher cognitive functions that developed much later from an evolutionary standpoint. Interestingly, it's the older parts of our brain, the brainstem and emotional center, that light up on brain scans. This indicates that stories are universal because they're actually hard-wired into our brain. This makes sense—after all, before humans could write, we needed a way to transmit information verbally in a memorable fashion. Stories are much easier to remember than a bunch of facts.[1]

Comedy is all about relating a story. A sketch is a well-prepared, thought-out story. An improv scene is a spur-of-the-moment story. A stand-up act is a succinct story, often told with just a few words. For a story to succeed, it needs to be in a language its audience can understand. In medicine, for a story to be understood by a patient in a clinical office setting, it should be jargon-free and in conversational tone. The story must also be the right length. If a sketch, improv scene, or stand-up act goes on too long, it loses its power. If a story to help a patient understand a concept goes on too long, the patient will stop paying attention. Stories help to educate patients in ways they can relate to.

Presence

Presence means to exist in the present moment. Presence can embody action or simply being.

When improvising or doing stand-up, you have to be in the present moment to succeed in connecting with the audience. Not only do you have to perform, you also have to listen to the audience—and not just to their words. You need to observe body language and facial expressions.

You have to react to the audience's feedback in real time. You can perform the exact same improvisation scene or stand-up act at two different times and get two completely different sets of audience feedback.

The comedian must be spontaneously creative and highly aware of the context. Otherwise, the audience will lose the connection and stop paying attention.

For patients and physicians to truly connect, the physician needs to be fully present in the moment, really listen to the patient by observing body language and facial expression. In paying attention to all of these factors, the physician can fully connect with the patient and also effectively react to the patient's feedback in real time. Being fully present allows the physician to be aware of the contextual nature of the visit and to spontaneously re-adjust as needed. For example, when discussing a medication change, the patient with a nervous eye flutter needs to be treated differently from the patient with a confident smile. Paying attention to these subtle cues can signal for the physician the best way to present the treatment plan.

Engagement

Engagement is about being interested in a task, issue, or event. In his classic TED talk, Simon Sinek discusses the power of why—in other words, purpose.[2] To really engage patients, you have to speak to their why. Patients don't follow medical instructions simply because they're told to. If a patient isn't engaged in a medical treatment plan, they often won't follow through with it. They have to understand the purpose behind it. "Why should I follow this plan? What's in for me? How will it make things better for me?" Is their why to fit into a new dress? Watch their children graduate from college? Or simply to be healthy enough after retirement to take that great trip? The why is crucial in medical follow-through.

A comedian can have a great story and be absolutely present in the moment and the performance can still go downhill if the audience isn't engaged. Audiences are engaged when they're being inspired, entertained, or educated. And that is achieved through the successful application of story, presence, and engagement.

The Most Obvious is Often the Most Powerful

When you need to put a smile on your face, what do you do? All I have to do is watch dogs surfing or toddlers getting into mischief. Smiling is such a simple thing, yet it's often ignored in medicine. Frowns are the norm in the halls of a hospital or the offices of a medical clinic. Yes, medicine is no joking matter. Yes, we're dealing with serious medical conditions. Yes, people's lives are literally in our hands. But does that mean we can't crack a smile, laugh at a joke, or spread some humor?

Ironically, the kind of comedy that can create change is often rooted in darkness. A good example is Trevor Noah's book *Born a Crime*. Noah relates many hilarious stories of growing up in South Africa. Underneath the humor are depictions of the sometimes horrifying sins of apartheid.[3] Noah's stage performances also raise serious topics in a funny way. And he delivers his comedy with a smile. Noah knows that a simple smile can go a long way when it comes to connecting with your audience.

And a smile from a healthcare provider can go a long way

when it comes to connecting with patients. Smiles make us more human. We know this intuitively as children. Many of us lose the natural tendency to smile somewhere along the line in medical training. I didn't realize this until a patient once told me that she didn't understand why I looked so serious all the time.

By partaking in comedy, I brought laughter back into my repertoire. The laughs and smiles around me were infectious. As comedians know full well, "We will never know all the good a simple smile can do."[4]

13. JUMP. DANCE. TREASURE.

WHAT STARTED out as an experiment in writing ended up becoming a three-year journey into the world of comedy. Comedic improvisation has served the purpose of allowing me to be creative, have fun, and flex my self-awareness muscles.

Because of comedy, I learned again to jump, dance, and treasure.

Jump

Not many things seem that scary after you've improvised a scene about frolicking teacups or performed a stand-up act in front of an audience that looks at you as if you're wasting their time.

Comedy took me from a place of risk-averse reserve to one of exploration. It stretched me as if I were a rubber band. I was forever expanded in new and wonderful ways. Comedy taught me to jump into new experiences with open-minded excitement.

The first rule of medicine, do no harm, is a good rule to follow. After all, an internist shouldn't prescribe a medication that could cause negative side effects unless there's a good reason to do so. In being overly cautious, we physicians are exercising due diligence. But what about when this need to be overly cautious in our job spills over into our personal lives, preventing us from trying new things that might result in experiencing joy?

Comedy has helped me be less mechanical and staid, more open to change.

Dance

I might as well have been dancing up on that improv stage, in fact on occasion I was. I could only do that because comedy taught me to be joyfully present: lessons that have carried over into my daily life.

Whether I'm there physically or just mentally, I smell my mother's curry and I can also taste the spices on my lips. I see my father enjoying a movie across the room—and I can also feel the warmth of his smile. I hear the words of a song—and I can also feel the notes move through my body. That feeling of carefree rebelliousness I get when I dance to my favorite song is now something I can feel whenever I'm joyfully present in the moment.

In delivering comedy, you use all five of your senses. You need to hear your scene partner's tone to react appropriately. You need to see if the audience is fidgeting or paying rapt attention to your jokes. You need to smell whether the audience has had a lot to drink, as this will impact their reaction to your jokes. You need to taste the air to determine the temperature—a cold audience will likely be a bit stiff. You need to feel your heartbeat to gauge how comfortable you are. No matter what information your senses feed you in the moment, you need to be positive to get through your comedy routine.

Comedy forces you to be joyfully present. If you perform stand-up comedy while not fully present, the audience can sense the lack of feeling in your words. You cannot read the audience or react to their input. And the very nature of improvisational comedy requires you to be present, as you make it up on the spot.

Treasure

Comedy gave me self-compassion. Because it teaches self-awareness, it forced me to recognize the extent of my burnout. I was a shell of my former determined, passionate self. It also forced me to expose and give voice to the causes of my burnout.

The best comedic material comes from authentic, unique experiences. My years putting up with racist, misogynistic patients and overbearing, uncaring administrators became great fodder for my stand-up act. They also became subjects for my comedic writing.

I learned to treasure my value, my worth, my unique persona.

The Comedic Cure

As physicians, we have to face a mountain of negativity, from treating vulnerable patients with serious medical conditions, to dealing with onerous administrators enforcing inane regulations. This negativity can fester in our work life and seep into our personal life. It is insidious, insatiable, and often seems intractable.

In order to beat the negativity, you need to combine the ability to jump into new adventures (provided they don't require physical dexterity), dance joyfully in the present moment with all five senses engaged, and treasure your uniqueness through self-compassion.

Despite our best efforts, we cannot change the past and we cannot know the future. The only thing we have is today. If we infuse the actions we take today with hope and confidence, we increase the likelihood that tomorrow will be full of bright possibilities.

My journey through comedy brought delight back into my life through laughter. By breaking down the negativity, opening me up to joyfulness, and allowing me to take my love with me everywhere I went, comedy healed the healer.

14. A BEAUTIFUL GOODBYE

Every act of creation is first an act of destruction.

PABLO PICASSO

PITTER. Patter. Splat.
Pitter. Patter. Splat.
Pitter. Patter. Splat.

Pitter went the raindrops. Patter went the car wheels. Splat went the books onto the floor. It was a crisp winter day, and I was seeking refuge in the bookstore café and its cinnamon-bun aroma. While perusing the travel section, I knocked over a stack of books. As I knelt to pick them up, one of them opened to a vintage cartoon of Popeye and Olive Oyl. In that moment, my world froze in guilt.

"You took the passing of my girl pretty hard."

I was transported back to the middle of my intern year. Transported back to Granny's death. The last time I'd seen Granddaddy was 5:16 a.m.

As 5:16 a.m. advanced to 4:12 p.m., the ICU printer was doing its best to get me home—by printing my sign-out sheet in shredded pieces. This particular printer had a reputation for moaning and groaning as though it were in competition with the actively laboring women in the maternity ward down the hall. And that afternoon, this printer gave birth to triplets.

As I battled the printer, Granddaddy tapped my shoulder. We sat down at a nurse's station, and he recalled his young-rascal days. Never in his wildest dreams had he thought he could get "such a beaut." But Granny was much more than a shore-leave beauty, and she'd honored this navy brat with over forty years of pearly white smiles, steely-toed support, and olive-eye gazes. He told me about a spinach-eating cartoon character named Popeye, whose girlfriend was called Olive Oyl. He wasn't sure when, but at some point in their marriage, Granny had become his Olive Oyl because of her olive-colored eyes. And Granddaddy had become her Popeye because of his spinach addiction.

As he reminisced, I witnessed a transformation in Granddaddy's sad eyes. First there were flickers, then embers, and then slowly but surely the fire of remembered passion re-ignited within his misty eyes.

At 6:37 p.m., another resident interrupted us and ordered me to go home. Granddaddy declared, "You took the passing of my girl pretty hard. I had over forty years of heaven with my girl. I figured, if you knew about our heaven, your day would get better."

Pitter. Patter. Splat.

Pitter. Patter. Splat.

Pitter. Patter. Splat.

Pitter went the shoes around me. Patter went the cutlery. Splat went the cake onto the floor. The splatter of the cake woke me out of my freeze, and in that moment, my world smiled. In that moment, I finally stopped focusing on Granny's death. I finally heard the extraordinary beauty within the ordinary destruction that had taken place that night. The beauty of Granny's butterfly-filled heart fluttering for her husband. The beauty of Granddaddy's comfort-filled words, meant to console my heart-ache. The beauty of Granddaddy's sincere devotion to his girl, and his saluting over forty years of heaven with Granny.

When we pluck a flower's petals, we cannot appreciate the flower. When we pluck away at life by focusing on the negativity, we cannot appreciate the beautiful moments—especially those incredible moments that shine brightly within the darkest hours.

As physicians, we hear about so much negativity in the lives of our patients. And the mess of our medical system and the daily practice of medicine itself can make us wonder if there's any beauty around us at all.

That morning in the bookstore, I stopped plucking and started listening—listening to the whispers of extraordinary beauty in everyday life. It was the moment I decided to seek answers outside traditional medicine. The moment that I started meandering. The moment that led me into the world of comedy, which healed me.

You have a choice. Hear the beauty. Instead of standing idly by, do something. Reframe the negativity. Adjust your situation to avoid the negativity. Or remove yourself from the situation to replace the negativity.

And if worse comes to worst, you can start from scratch. Destroy the situation. Destroy the negativity. Destroy the burn-out. Don't be afraid to destroy the status quo.

You have a choice. Hear the beauty—the beauty within the destruction.

Now, when I look back at Granny' death, at 3:48 a.m., I stop plucking. I start listening. I see the beauty of Granddaddy's wrinkled hands pulling Granny's eyelashes over her olive eyes. I hear his words of devotion saluting over forty years of marriage. I know the love in his fluttering heart is hers forever.

In that moment of goodbye, ordinary life whispered extraordinary beauty.

It was, it still is, and it will forever be a most beautiful destruction.

APPENDIX

If you're interested in trying your hand at improvisation, stand-up comedy, or comedic writing, here are a few useful sites:

1. Improvisation: improvencyclopedia.org/games/. This site includes a list of improv games you can try with your friends for free.
2. Stand-up comedy: https://standupny.teachable.com/. This site offers online stand-up comedy classes.
3. Comedic writing: https://trainingcenter.secondcity.com/. No matter what type of comedic writing you're interested in (e.g., satire, sketch writing, etc.), The Second City offers great classes.

Most major cities have comedy clubs that offer classes in improv, stand- up, and comedic writing. And check out social media to find local comedy-writing organizations, improvisation jams, and stand-up comedy groups. I did not use social media beyond Facebook and Meetup.com. However, I've heard from local comedians that there are many comedy groups flourishing on different social media channels. These are good ways to get your feet wet without putting out too much money.

If this book sparked an interest in communication in general, I highly recommend Alan Alda's podcast *Clear+Vivid* (www.alda-communicationtraining.com/podcasts/). I could have filled this whole book with how the information shared in this podcast can be applied to medicine. As you can see, I restrained myself.

If you're a burned-out physician just looking for some laughs, I highly recommend Dr. Zubin Damania's musical parodies (https://zdoggmd.com/).

No matter which path you choose, I hope you take the leap into comedy.

Good luck on your adventure!

ACKNOWLEDGMENTS

It's impossible to thank everybody who inspired me along my comedy journey.

To the people whose names I've forgotten, please forgive me. Your help was invaluable.

Great thanks goes to the team who put this book together—Boni, John, and the team at Ingenium Books. I appreciate all that you've taught me.

Deep gratitude goes to all within the comedy community who taught me. This includes Allison, Stephanie, Improv Chris, Stand-Up Chris from the DC Improv, Caitlin from the Belladonna Comedy, Kathy and Shawn from the Unified Scene Theater, Kerby from the Arlington Public Library, and all the local comedians who helped me along my journey: Victoria, Suzie, Vicky, Bana, Kenneth, Haywood, Michelle, Gabriel, Jason, Angela, Hank, Brandon, J.J., Nick, Domnic, Kim, Jelani, and Gigi. Also thanks to the non-comedians who braved the comedy experiences with me: Vidhika, J.K., Mahesh, and Brian.

Eternal gratitude goes to all the friends and family who urged me along this journey and supported me through my comedic endeavors and the writing of this book. Very special thanks goes out to Mahesh, Sowmya, Mani, Praveen, Raja, Pradeep, Thanhvan, Karen, Heidi, Margaret, Tam-Chinh, Laura, Stewie, Kylan, Tina, Aimee, Swathi, Priya, and Ellen.

Most of all, thank you Mom and Dad—without both of you, I'm nothing.

And if you've read this far, I thank you, the reader, for the gift of your time.

Please take a moment now and leave a review where you purchased this book. Reader reviews are very, very important to independent authors like me, as they are the best way to help other readers decide whether the book is right for them. So, please leave a review for this book. I will be extremely grateful. Thank you.

ABOUT THE AUTHOR

Pranathi Kondapaneni is a physician, writer, and explorer-in-chief. At the age of sixteen, she was accepted into a combined BA/ MD program. By the age of twenty-four, she had completed four degrees: two undergraduate degrees (economics and biology), a master's in public health, and a medical degree. After completing a residency in neurology and two fellowships in sleep and epilepsy, Dr. Kondapaneni went on to become a private-practice attending physician for a decade.

Due to her frustration with clinical medicine, in 2015 Dr. Kondapaneni set out on a series of adventures to help improve communication in the medical office and combat physician burnout. These adventures have varied from comedy routines to classes on artistic visual observation. Dr. Kondapaneni enjoys exploring other disciplines in order to empower physicians to improve communication and combat burnout.

She lives in Michigan but has traveled to many countries, including Australia, India, Chile, and South Africa. She also likes traveling around the United States. She enjoys listening to audiobooks and podcasts, the smell of coffee in the a.m., sip-ping on a good cup of tea, and soaking up culture through art, architecture, food, or a great movie.

Connect with Pranathi:
https://ingeniumbooks.com/pranathi-kondapaneni/

OTHER BOOKS BY PRANATHI:

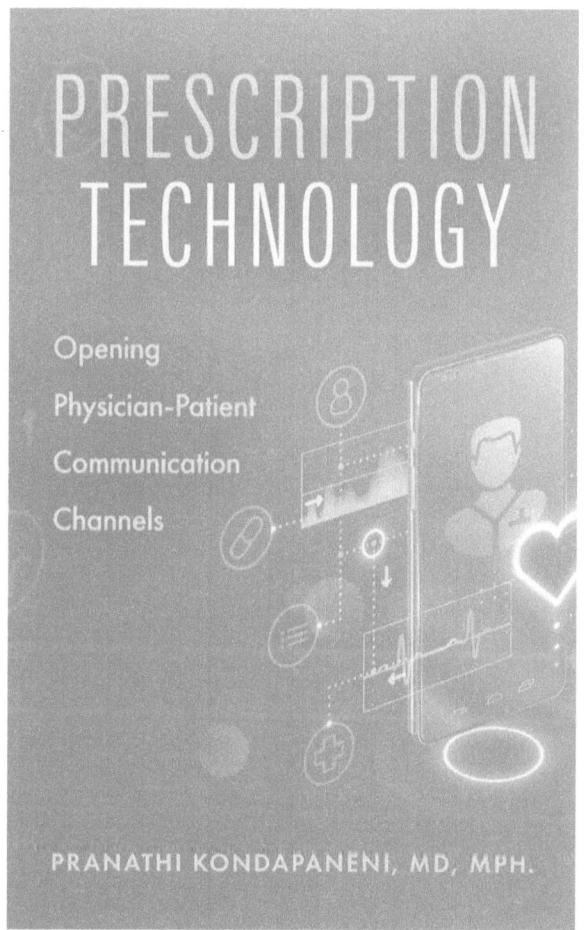

NOTES

Introduction

1. "Hippocratic Oath," Wikipedia, last modified January 5th, 2019, https://en.wikipedia.org/wiki/Hippocratic_Oath.

3. Anatomy of Physician Burnout

1. Zubin Damania, Are Zombie Doctors Taking Over America, video filmed April 2013 at TEDMED2013, Washington D.C., June 2013, https://zdoggmd.com/tedmed/.
2. Medscape National Physician and Burnout Report 2018, Survey posted January 17, 2018, https://www.medscape.com/ slideshow/2018-lifestyle-burnout-depression-6009235.
3. Christina Maslach, Michael P. Leiter, The Truth About Burnout: How Organizations Cause Personal Stress and What to Do About It, San Francisco, California, Jossey-Bass, 1997, 14.
4. Medscape National Physician and Burnout Report 2018.
5. Pamela Wible, "Why Doctors Kill Themselves," Filmed November 2015, TEDMED2015, Palm Springs, California, Video posted March 2016, https://www.tedmed.com/talks/ show?id=528918.

4. Female Physician Burnout

1. I. Houkes, Y. Winants, M. Twellaar, P. Verdonk, "Development of Burn-out Over Time and the Causal Order of the Three Dimensions of Burnout Among Male and Female GPs, A Three-Wave Panel Study," BMC Public Health, 11 (2011), 240.
2. "MomMD," Accessed January 8th, 2019, https://www. mommd.com/.

6. The Burnout Cure

1. RuthAnn Richter, "In a First for Academic Medical Center, Stanford Hires Chief Wellness Officer," Stanford Medical News Center, June 22, 2017, https://med.stanford.edu/news/ all-news/2017/06/stanford-medicine-hires-chief-physician-wellness-officer.html.

2. "The First Conference on Physician Health at Stanford," Accessed January 8th, 2019, wellmd.stanford.edu/content/ dam/sm/wellmd/documents/2017-ACPH-pub.pdf.
3. "The Happy MD," Accessed January 8th, 2019, https://www.thehappymd.com/.
4. Michael Lee, "Michael Lee of Kaiser Permanente," interviewed by Thomas Yoon, Yoon Know What, Season 2, Episode 3, Youtube Video, Posted on January 9th, 2019.

7. The Flame Challenge

1. "The Flame Challenge," Accessed January 8th, 2019, https:// www.aldacenter.org/outreach/flame-challenge.
2. "Alan Alda," Wikipedia, last modified January 8th, 2019, https://en.wikipedia.org/wiki/Alan_Alda.
3. The Flame Challenge.

9. The Connection Conundrum

1. Mick Napier, Improvise-Scene from the Inside Out, Denver, Merriweather Publishing, 2015, 1.
2. Alan Alda, If I Understood You, Would I Have This Look on My Face? My Adventures in the Art and Science of Relating and Communicating, (New York: Random House, 2017), 50-51.
3. "The 7 Habits of Highly Effective People," Wikipedia, modified January 5th, 2019, https://en.wikipedia.org/wiki/ The_7_Habits_of_Highly_Effective_People.

10. Foreign Accents

1. "Haywood Turnipseed Jr," Accessed January 8th, 2019, haywoodturnipseedjr.com/.

11. Educate, Entertain, Inspire

1. Shonda Rhimes, "My Year of Saying Yes to Everything," Filmed February 2016, TED2016, Vancouver, British Columbia, Canada, Video posted February 2016, https://www.ted.com/talks/shonda_rhimes_my_year_of_saying_yes_to_everything?...en.
2. "Scrubs," Wikipedia, modified January 5th, 2019, https:// en.wikipedia.org/wiki/Scrubs_(TV_series).
3. Caitlin Kunkel, "I Ate a Sweet Potato for Breakfast and Now I'm a Fitness Celebrity," The Belladonna, December 6th, 2018, https://

thebelladonnacomedy.com/i-ate-a-sweet-potato-for-breakfast-and-now-im-a-fitness-celebrity-c6e89c9ed9e8.
4. Joanna Penn, "5 Tips For Successful Publishing and Book Marketing Lessons Learned From the Independent Author Conference." The Creative Penn Podcast, Episode 402, Audio podcast, November 12th, 2018, https://www.thecreativepenn. com/2018/11/12/5-tips-for-successful-publishing-and-book-marketing-lessons-learned-from-the-independent-author-conference/.
5. "First Year Funk-An Uptown Funk Parody by Wash U St. Louis School of Medicine," WUSM2018 YouTube channel, published May 10th, 2015, https://www.youtube.com/ watch?v=2q1kQRmzIaY.
6. "Let Me Go ['Let It Go' Frozen Med School Parody]," UMDSOM2015 YouTube channel, published July 12th, 2014, https://www.youtube.com/watch?v=7Y53Yd01zJw.
7. Zdoggmd, "Can't Feel My Face," Video published February 24th, 2016, https://zdoggmd.com/cant-feel-my-face/.
8. Zdoggmd, "EHR State of Mind," Video published October 19th, 2015, https://zdoggmd.com/ehr-state-of-mind/.

12. The Good of a Simple Smile

1. Jonathan Gottschall, The Storytelling Animal: How Stories Make Us Human, Boston: Mariner Books, April 13th, 2013, 36-82.
2. Simon Sinek, "How Great Leaders Inspire Action," Filmed September 2009 at TEDx Puget Sound, Washington, Video posted, May 2010, https://www.ted.com/speakers/simon_ sinek.
3. Trevor Noah, Born a Crime: Stories from a South African Childhood. Ch 1-3, Grand Haven, Michigan, Brilliance Audio: November 15th, 2016, Audiobook, https://www. brillianceaudio.com/product?i=29063.
4. Bert Jacobs, John Jacobs, Life Is Good: Simple Words from Jake And Rocket, New York: Meredith Books, 2007.

www.ingramcontent.com/pod-product-compliance
Lightning Source LLC
Chambersburg PA
CBHW021449070526
44577CB00002B/321